Dance Your Way Into Better Fitness and Health with Nutritional Harmony

Table of Contents

Chapter 1. Introduction

Dive into a vibrant world of rhythmic beats and wholesome bites with our Special Report, "Dance Your Way Into Better Fitness and Health with Nutritional Harmony". This cheerfully engaging guide invites you – regardless of your previous dance or dietary experiences – to embark on a thrilling journey towards improved wellbeing. We fuse together the sheer joy of dancing with the science of nutrition, creating an enjoyable pathway to enhanced fitness and health that will keep you tapping your feet while fueling them right. The upbeat nature of this Special Report is sure to inspire you, engendering an eagerness to explore the manifold benefits of combining rhythmical movement with balanced nutrition. By the end of this paragraph, we bet you'll be ready to grab your dancing shoes and grocery list to begin your delightful journey into better health with our Special Report!

Chapter 2. Dance Basics: Understanding the Rhythm of Your Health

Before we delve into understanding the rhythm of your health, roll up your sleeves and loosen the knots in your brain because this is where we plant seeds of health and fitness wisdom into the soil of your intellectual garden.

First things first - let's understand the core principle; every individual has a unique rhythm, a unique beat their body moves to, and understanding this beat requires our deepest attention. This rhythm is your personalized approach to dance and fitness. Coupling this rhythm with nutritional harmony can lead to a boost in health, performance, and overall quality of life.

Now, let's embark on this invigorating journey with basic dance knowledge.

2.1. Understanding Dance as Exercise

For time immortal, dance has been one of the most expressive forms of art and communication. Yet, when it comes to fitness, dance is often overlooked. It is important to consider dance as not just an art form, but also recognize it as a very comprehensive form of physical exercise that engages the whole body. Essentially, it is cardio exercise that offers the added benefits of strength training, flexibility, endurance, and balance.

A dance routine can burn as many calories as jogging, swimming, or cycling. The calorie-burning aspect of dance significantly depends on

"

the intensity, style, duration, and your personal effort. From the energetic beats of Zumba to the slow and controlled movements of ballet, each dance genre offers different health benefits and engages different muscle groups.

2.2. Importance of Rhythm in Dance

Rhythm is a principal element in dance. It is the pattern of regular or irregular pulses caused in music by the occurrence of strong and weak melodic and harmonic beats. Understanding the rhythm helps you connect with the music, guide your bodily movements, and maintain a steady pace. This is similar to understanding your body rhythm for a healthier life.

The flow of energy in the body, your mood swings, hunger patterns, sleep, heart rate, even your feelings of fatigue and alertness, contribute to your internal body rhythm or biological rhythm. Aligning these rhythms with your dance routine and diet can be a game-changer for health optimization. Just as rhythm is key to dancing, it is crucial to synchronize the rhythm of what you eat, how much, and when – to achieve the best state of health.

2.3. How to Find Your Dance Rhythm

Finding your dance rhythm can be a phenomenally personal and liberating experience. Start slow, let your body acquaint itself with the very basic steps. Try some basic steps from genres like Ballroom, Hip Hop, Contemporary, or even Street Dance. Gradually increase the intensity of movements. It's like tuning a radio to find the correct frequency, fine-tuning your movements will allow you to understand your body's rhythm better.

Use mirrors extensively. Visual feedback can be your greatest critic and strongest aid in your dance journey. Observing yourself will not only help enhance your movements but also boost your confidence in your dance capabilities.

2.4. Understanding Your Nutrition Needs

Just as movement varies from person to person, so do nutritional needs. Understanding the dynamics of your body's requirements is pivotal to ensure your diet nurtures your health and sustains your dance routine.

Evaluate your lifestyle and your body's need for nutrients, factoring in gender, age, level of activity, and any specific health condition(s). A balanced diet, rich in macronutrients (proteins, fats, carbohydrates) and micronutrients (vitamins, minerals), combined with adequate hydration, nurtures the body, fuels the dance, and aids faster recovery.

2.5. Combining Dance and Nutrition

Synchronizing dance with balanced nutrition could be likened to a perfectly choreographed ballet. Each nourishing bite guides your body seamlessly through the rhythm of your dance routine. The harmony maximizes energy utilization and boosts recovery, keeping you moving to the beat with utmost confidence and strength.

Remember, food is fuel, but it takes a specific balance to keep things running smoothly. Take a cue from professional dancers – their diets often consist of lean proteins for muscle repair and recovery, complex carbohydrates for sustained energy, and healthy fats for prolonged satiety.

2.6. Conclusion

Understanding this rhythm, your very own rhythm, will guide you down the path of dancing to the melodies of health, fitness, and happiness.

Embrace the rhythm of dance, embrace the rhythm of health, create your harmony with the best of food and dance. Use this chapter as a guide – but ultimately, let your body guide you in this dance of life on the stage of health. This rhythm is yours, and when you feel it deep within, let it fuel not just your dance but your life with the pure emotion of happiness and satisfaction of achieving health through dance. Remember, you're one dance away from a good mood!

Grasp your dancing shoes, sway with the rhythm, and dance your way into better health. Conclude your dance sessions with wholesome bites, and experience a transcendent journey towards enhanced fitness, health, and overall wellbeing.

Chapter 3. Decoding Nutrition: Foods That Fuel Your Dance

Just as how it's essential to know your dance moves, understanding what fuels your body for those movements is equally vital. Nutrition is the cornerstone of physical performance and dance is no exception. Let's explore some key components that will enhance your overall dancing capability and performance.

3.1. What is Nutrition?

Nutrition is the science that investigates the relationship between diet and health. It primarily focuses on the dietary needs of an organism to stay healthy and functional. Good nutrition, therefore, means eating a diet rich in essential nutrients which include proteins, carbohydrates, fats, vitamins, and minerals, all of which play vital roles in our body's function, growth, and maintenance.

3.2. Role of Nutrition in Dance

Engaging in dance places a substantial demand on your body. Therefore, it is essential to fuel your body with an appropriate mix of macronutrients (proteins, carbohydrates, and fats) and micronutrients (vitamins and minerals) to accommodate these demands.

In dance, the body functions as an integrated entity, seeking energy from various dietary sources to support an array of physical tasks. Nutrients serve both as a fuel to energize you and as construction materials necessary for repairing and building new tissues. Hence, proper nutrition helps improve muscular strength, increase aerobic and anaerobic power, and enhance overall performance.

3.3. Proteins: Building Blocks for Your Dance

Proteins, often classified as the building blocks of life, are essential for our bodies. They're responsible for muscle development, strength, and recovery which are crucial points for a dancer.

Meat, fish, eggs, and dairy products are excellent sources of animal protein. For those who have a plant-based diet, options include beans, lentils, chickpeas, and tofu. Remember, protein is not just about quantity, but also about quality—make sure you have a variety of protein sources to get all Essential Amino Acids.

3.4. Carbohydrates: Fuel for Your Rhythm

Carbohydrates are your body's primary energy source. They are broken down by your body into glucose, which is used to fuel your muscles during dance. Hence, consuming the right amount and type of carbohydrates is essential.

Whole grains, fruits, and vegetables are rich in carbohydrates, offering a steady supply of energy instead of sharp peaks and declines that come from refined carbs found in candies and soft drinks. As a dancer, it's recommended to consume complex carbohydrates like cereals, whole grain bread and pasta.

3.5. Fats: Don't Shy Away

For long, fats have been unduly vilified. However, it's important to understand that not all fats are created equal. While trans fats and some saturated fats are harmful, unsaturated fats, particularly omega-3 fatty acids, are essential for overall health.

Fats assist in energy production, absorption of fat-soluble vitamins, and cushioning of vital organs. Excellent sources of healthy fats include avocados, nuts, seeds, olives, and fatty fish.

3.6. Hydration: The Lifeline

Hydration is vital to dancers, mainly because dancing is an intense physical activity that causes sweating. Dehydration can result in a decrease in performance, concentration, and increased fatigue.

Water is an excellent hydration source, but in high-intensity dance sessions, you may require a sports drink containing essential electrolytes lost through sweat.

3.7. Vitamins and Minerals: Tiny Components, Big Impact

Lastly, vitamins and minerals, although required in small amounts, play critical roles in energy production, hemoglobin synthesis, bone health, and immune function. Again, a diet rich in various colored vegetables, fruits, whole grains, lean proteins, and healthy fats usually provides an adequate supply of these essential micronutrients.

3.8. Dancer's Plate: A Sample Meal Plan

Here is a sample meal plan that fuels the dancing body:

- **Breakfast**: Oatmeal with fruits, nuts, and a scoop of protein powder.

- **Mid-Morning Snack**: Greek yogurt with a handful of almonds.

- **Lunch**: Grilled chicken with mixed vegetables and quinoa.

- **Afternoon Snack**: A piece of dark chocolate and an apple.

- **Dinner**: Baked salmon, sweet potato, and green salad.

- **Evening Snack:** Cottage cheese and berries.

These meals offer a balanced mix of macro and micronutrients that are essential for a dancer's body.

This journey into nutritive harmony is all about balance – balancing the right quality and quantity of food to complement your dance. By ingesting the right kinds of nutrients in adequate amounts, you are providing your body with the necessary fuel it needs to dance with grace, strength, and passion. The process might seem daunting at first, but remember, every good journey starts with a single step. So, let's take that step towards better dance performance and overall health today!

Chapter 4. Step-by-Step: Aligning Dance Moves with Nutritional Needs

Dancing can be an exceptional tool for physical fitness, but coupling it with the power of nutrition can truly elevate one's health. This chapter is essentially crafted to guide you through marrying dance movements with nutritional needs, aiming to provide a comprehensive package for better well-being.

Before we delve into specific dance moves and coordinating nutritional requirements, there are a few key principles to understand. Dance is a full-body workout, taxing both aerobic and anaerobic systems. Different kinds of dance place different demands on the body, but all require energy, hydration, and a balance of macro and micronutrients. Paying attention to specific nutrient needs based on your dance routine can help you recover faster, build strength, and dance longer.

4.1. Establishing Your Nutritional Foundation

To begin the journey towards combining dance with nutrition, one must first create a sound nutritional foundation. A balanced diet consists of the right mix of macronutrients – proteins, carbohydrates, fats – and micronutrients – vitamins, minerals. In the context of dance, these will refuel your body and help it repair itself, aiding in performance enhancement and injury prevention.

Carbohydrates, for instance, are essential for energy. As you dance, your body breaks down carbohydrates into glucose, supplying immediate energy, and glycogen, reserved for later use. Proteins, on the other hand, repair the muscle damage incurred during a dance session, while fats provide long-term energy and aid in nutrient absorption.

Equally important are the micronutrients derived from a balanced diet. Iron, for instance, helps transport oxygen from lungs to muscles, while calcium and vitamin D promote strong bones, reducing the risk of stress fractures common in dancers.

4.2. Identifying Dance-Specific Nutritional Needs

Dance forms like ballet, jazz, tap, or hip-hop come with their specific dietary requirements. For instance, ballet is traditionally anaerobic, requiring quick bursts of energy supplied by glycogen reserves. Eating a diet rich in complex carbohydrates will help fill these reserves, empowering ballet dancers to leap, turn, and glide on stage.

Hip hop and tap dance, contrastingly, are more aerobic, requiring steady energy production. A slow-release energy source is best met through balanced meals composed of proteins, complex carbohydrates, and healthy fats eaten at regular intervals.

4.3. Creating a Nutrition Plan

A successful nutrition plan aligns with dance timings, load, and intensity. Pre-dance meals should aim to provide immediate energy through simple carbohydrates, while post-dance meals should focus on replenishing glycogen reserves and promoting muscle recovery with a mix of complex carbohydrates, proteins, and some fats.

Additionally, having small but nutrient-dense snacks for slow-release energy during longer dance practices can keep fatigue at bay and sustain concentration.

A sample nutrition plan for a day of intense dance might include:

- A pre-dance breakfast of whole-grain cereal with milk
- A mid-morning snack of nuts and dried fruits
- A balanced lunch of fish or tofu, brown rice and veggies
- A pre-dinner, post-practice snack of Greek yogurt with berries
- A dinner featuring lean protein, roasted vegetables and quinoa
- A late-night snack of wholegrain toast with nut butter

This is simply a guide and individual needs may vary. It's also essential to integrate hydration into your nutrition plan – aim to consume at least two liters of water throughout the day, with additional fluids if dancing intensely.

4.4. Adapting Nutritional Needs to Dance Progression

As you progress in your dance journey, your dietary needs will evolve. Increased fitness levels will agilely decrease your body's glycogen usage, meaning you will extract more energy from less food. But as dance routines become more advanced and intense, the demand for nutrients to repair and build muscles will increase.

It's crucial, therefore, to periodically reevaluate your nutrition plan, considering changing dance loads and intensities. Testing different food timings, quantities, and combinations on practice days can help fine-tune what works best for your body.

Always remember, through combining rhythmic dance moves and fundamental nutrition, we have the opportunity to tap into a joyous and active pursuit of improved health. Pairing the physicality of dance with the science of nutrition creates a harmonious alliance that truly lets you "dance your way" into better fitness and health.

Chapter 5. Energy in Motion: Balancing Caloric Intake with Dance Routines

Focusing on energy in motion and the balance of caloric intake with dance, we have to start where it all begins: the calories themselves. Calories are essentially a measure of energy, vital to our daily functioning. It's the fuel your body uses to perform all activities, from complex cognitive processes to simple physical movements.

5.1. Understanding Calories

A calorie is a unit of energy that measures how much energy food provides to the body. The body has a certain caloric need to perform its basic functions, known as basal metabolic rate (BMR), but the type, intensity, and length of physical activities also significantly contribute to the total energy expenditure. To maintain a healthy weight and overall wellness, it's important to balance the calories you consume from foods with the calories you expend during daily physical activity.

5.2. Why Dance?

Dance is hailed not only as an art form and a means of self-expression but also as an excellent way to burn calories. Regardless of the form—be it Zumba, ballet, salsa, or hip-hop—dancing elevates your heart rate, tones your muscles, and torches calories. For someone weighing around 155 pounds, a 30-minute dance session can burn between 130-250 calories, depending on the intensity and type of dance. The great thing about dance is it's an all-in-one activity that combines cardiovascular exercise, strength work, and flexibility, all while fun rhythms set an upbeat tempo.

5.3. Know Your Dance Forms

Every dance style has a different intensity and will lead to a different caloric burn rate. For example, moderate-intensity dances like ballroom dance might burn approximately 219 calories per hour whereas high-intensity dance forms like Zumba can incinerate up to 446 calories in an hour! Considering these differences is important when planning a dance-fitness regimen that targets a specific caloric goal.

5.4. Caloric Balance and Dance

Everyone has a unique caloric balance that consists of the calories consumed versus the calories burned. To maintain your current weight, these two should typically be equal; to lose weight, you need to burn more calories than consumed. This is another area where dance steps in—as a delightful and enjoyable way, not only to balance, but to tip the scales in favor of calorie burn. Yet, it's important not to compensate for the extra burned calories by consuming more than your body needs.

5.5. Balanced Diet for Dancing

Dancing is a physical activity that requires energy. Consuming the right type and amount of food can provide you with this energy. Here, the interplay between macronutrients - carbohydrates, proteins, and fats - becomes crucial.

- Carbohydrates: They are dancers' main energy source. Complex carbohydrates like whole grains, fruits, and vegetables provide sustained energy and should make up around 55%-60% of a dancer's diet.

- Proteins: Necessary for muscle recovery and repair. Include lean meats, eggs, and legumes in your diet.

- Fats: Needed for energy and absorption of certain vitamins. Healthy fats can be found in foods such as avocados, nuts, seeds, and oily fish.

5.6. Calorie Counting and Dancing

Keeping track of the calories you consume from your diet and burn during your dance exercises can ensure you're maintaining a balance. Create a chart detailing your calorie consumption and burn rate. Calculating this regularly can help you adjust your dance routine and diet accordingly to meet your health goals.

Nutrition labels found on packaged foods can be helpful. They list the calorie content per serving, along with other important information, such as fat, carbohydrate, and protein content. There are also numerous online tools and apps that can help you track calories consumed and burned.

5.7. Meeting Hydration Needs

Maintaining hydration is vital as the body loses water and electrolytes during dancing through sweat. Although not a direct component of calorie balance, hydration aids in digestion and nutrient assimilation, indirectly impacting your overall caloric balance. It's advised to consume small quantities of water throughout the dance session and have a larger amount post-session to replenish the lost fluids.

5.8. Conclusion

The harmony between dance and a balanced diet provides a fun, but effective, approach to fitness and health. By understanding your caloric needs, choosing the right dance forms, maintaining a balanced diet, and monitoring the caloric intake and burn, you can effectively harness the joy of dance to serve your health goals. Dance your way to health, but remember, the journey is as significant, if not more, than the destination. So, savor every movement, every beat, and every bite!

Chapter 6. Culture Explosion: Traditional Dances and their Nutritional Complements

Just as you cannot separate the vibrant rhythms from a flamenco performance or the graceful leaps from a ballet, dance and the culture from which it emerges are inseparable. The types of movements, the music, even the costumes, are all deeply influenced by the cultural heritage and history of a dance. But what's often overlooked are the traditional diets that fuel these incredible performances.

With this in mind, let's dive into a world tour of traditional dances and the food that nourishes the dancers.

6.1. Ballroom Dance and English Cuisine

Infused with elegance and rigorous techniques, Ballroom dance is a formal style of social dancing, dating back to the 16th century. The strenuous training requires a lot of energy, and the quintessential diet of English people provides just that. Their diet traditionally consists of hearty ingredients, high in proteins and carbohydrates, like various kinds of meats, potatoes, and dairy products. This allows dancers to continually replenish their energy.

One classic dish is the Shepherd's Pie, a comforting, healthy meal packed with lamb or beef, mixed vegetables, and a top layer of mashed potatoes. This high-protein, high-carb dish effectively fuels the strenuous footwork, twirls, and lifts common in Ballroom dancing.

6.2. Flamenco and Mediterranean Diet

Birthed in the Andalusian region of Spain, Flamenco is a passionate dance form that's as much about the rhythm as it is about the dancer's emotional expression. Flamenco dancers often follow a Mediterranean diet, known for its heart-healthy benefits.

The staples of a Mediterranean diet include fresh fruits, vegetables, lean proteins, and heart-healthy fats - like those found in olive oil and fish. Staple dishes like Paella, a flavorful mix of saffron rice, various seafood, meat, and colorful vegetables provide dancers with slow-releasing energy.

6.3. Hula Dance and Hawaiian Diet

Hawaiian Hula dancers use every part of their bodies to tell a story. The mesmerizing dance form needs energized bodies that Hawaiian traditional diet rich in fresh fruits, fish, and local vegetables can provide.

Poi, a nutritious staple made from taro, provides valuable nutrients including Vitamin C, fiber, and necessary carbohydrates. Mixed with fresh, vibrant fruits like mango and pineapple, this diet not only satiates the appetite but provides a long-lasting energy supply.

6.4. Kathak Dance and Indian Nutrition

Kathak, one of the most distinguished Indian classical dances, demands agility, strength, and grace. It can be extensive, and as such, dancers require diets that aid stamina. Indian diets, rich in fibrous vegetables, lentils, grains, fruits with a fair amount of dairy, and spices, make for a balanced, energizing diet.

A dancer's meal could be something as simple and nutritious as Khichdi (a blend of lentils and rice) combined with yogurt and salad. Highly versatile, this meal can be adjusted with more vegetables or lean meats, as per the individual's nutritional requirements.

6.5. Capoeira and Brazilian Cuisine

Capoeira is not just a dance form but also a martial art that requires quick, high-energy movements. Brazilian cuisine, aligned perfectly with these needs, is a colorful blend of corn, beans, meat, and tropical fruits.

Feijoada, a black bean stew with various cuts of meat served with rice, greens and orange slices, is a typical Brazilian dish. This protein-packed meal keeps Capoeira dancers moving swiftly, enabling their acrobatic kicks and airborne maneuvers.

Through this exploration of five different dance styles and their corresponding traditional diets, we see a common thread. Each culture's gastronomical offerings align beautifully with the energy requirements of their traditional dances. Plus, relying on the whole, minimally processed foods native to their regions provides dancers with a myriad of health benefits beyond fuel for their dancing.

This fusion of culture, dance, and nutrition shows us how intertwined these aspects of a healthy lifestyle are. Furthermore, it offers insight into how maintaining a balance of physical activity with appropriate, culturally-anchored nutrition can lead us to a healthier, more energetic life. No matter where you come from or what style of dance you practice, eating a balanced diet from a variety of food sources is key to powering your dance steps and maintaining your overall health.

Chapter 7. Beyond Calories: Embracing Micronutrients in Your Dance Diet

When we talk about nutrition, often the first thing that comes to mind are calories. While counting calories can be important, it's only part of the story regarding what your body needs. To truly embrace a healthy diet that complements your dance regimen and improves your overall fitness, we need to look beyond just the calories and delve into the world of micronutrients.

7.1. Understanding Micronutrients

Rather than being direct sources of energy, like carbohydrates, proteins, and fats, micronutrients are those vital vitamins and minerals that regulate your body's various processes. They're called 'micro' because your body requires them in lesser quantities, but their effects on your health are anything but small!

When dancing, your body goes through rigorous physical activity and loses not only calories but these essential micronutrients too. They need to be replenished for proper body function, for improving your dance performance, and for a holistic approach to health.

7.2. The Importance of Vitamins

Vitamins are organic compounds needed by the body in small amounts for various roles, from forming bones, healthy skin, and blood cells to supporting the nervous system and the immune system responses.

For dancers specifically, vitamins C and E are critical as they serve as antioxidants that reduce muscle damage. Vitamin D is essential for bone strength as dancers put much pressure on their skeletal system during performances. The B-vitamins play a crucial part in energy production and muscle repair. For example, niacin (Vitamin B3) helps breakdown and use fats and carbohydrates for energy during dance sessions.

7.3. Enriching Minerals

Like vitamins, minerals play an essential role in the proper functioning of the body. For a dancer, calcium and magnesium are vital for bone health and muscle contraction, respectively. Iron aids in the transport of oxygen to muscles during dance routines, while zinc helps with the healing of any injuries and boosts the immune system.

Keep in mind that while minerals are crucial, they should be balanced. Overconsumption can interfere with the body's ability to absorb other minerals.

7.4. Making Your Plate Colorful

To keep up with the needs of dancers, meals should consist of a variety of colorful fruits and vegetables. Think dark greens such as spinach and Swiss chard, vibrant oranges and yellows like bell peppers, pumpkin, sweet potatoes, and bright blues and purples found in blueberries and beetroot. These foods are brimming with a vast array of micronutrients, from vitamin C in citrus fruits to Magnesium in dark greens and the lutein in bright orange veggies.

7.5. Micronutrients and Energy

Micronutrients don't directly supply energy in the way macronutrients do, but being deficient in them can certainly affect your energy levels and dance performance. B-vitamins, for example, are important in converting macronutrients into usable energy. An inadequate intake could result in fatigue and a reduced ability to focus on your dance routines.

7.6. Comprehensive Micronutrient Sources

Aside from fruits and vegetables, whole grains, lean protein, and dairy products also contain a ton of essential micronutrients. Opt for whole grains like brown rice, oatmeal, and quinoa that are rich in magnesium, iron, and B-vitamins. Lean proteins such as fish, chicken, and turkey are packed with iron and B-vitamins. Dairy products like milk and cheese are excellent sources of calcium and vitamin D.

7.7. Positive Hydration Habits

Hydration is another important aspect that must be considered. Dancers lose a lot of body water through intense dance workouts. It's vital to replenish not only the fluids but also the minerals, notably electrolytes (such as sodium, potassium, and magnesium), which are lost through sweat.

7.8. Avoiding Micronutrient Deficiencies

A lack of any micronutrient can negatively impact your health and performance. Possible signs can range from fatigue and reduced immune functioning to more serious problems such as anemia caused by iron deficiency or even scurvy due to a lack of vitamin C!

To ensure you are getting an adequate amount of these critical nutrients, consider consulting with a dietitian who can analyze your diet and give you a plan suitable for your dancing regimen and general health status.

7.9. Tailoring Your Diet

Every dancer's body is unique, and their needs can vary significantly. Factors like the dance genre, number of hours you dance, recovery time, and your personal goals all play a part in determining how much and what kind of micronutrients you need. Working with a dietitian can help tailor a plan to meet your personal needs.

7.10. Conclusion

Attention to micronutrients in your dance diet can be a game changer, improving your dance prowess, reducing injury likelihood, and promoting overall health. Understanding and incorporating the right amount of micronutrients into your diet can make the path to better health not just a dance, but a joyous and colorful performance that you enjoy daily!

Chapter 8. Mastering Hydration: Your Best Dance Partner

In the world of dance, rhythm and pace set the stage. But what truly powers the performance is not merely the prowess of the dancer or the right choice of music. It is something much more elemental, something as essential as water. Yes, we're talking about hydration, your unheralded dance partner in the pursuit of better health and fitness.

8.1. How Important is Hydration?

It's no understatement to proclaim hydration as life-sustaining. Our bodies are approximately 60% water. This magical liquid doesn't just act as a building block for cells, it also lubricates joints, regulates body temperature, and aids digestion. Every single system in our body depends upon it.

For dancers, who expend energy in swathes and depend on optimum body functioning, hydration becomes even more crucial. Dancing, an activity involving extensive movements, leads to a significant loss of fluids through perspiration. Continuous dehydration can lead to decreased performance, muscle cramps, and, in worse scenarios, serious health implications such as heat strokes.

8.2. Know Your Hydration Levels

A key aspect of mastering hydration is simply being aware of your body's requirements. This hinges on understanding the telltale signs of dehydration. Too often, thirst isn't an adequate indicator, as you might already be dehydrated by the time you feel thirsty. Look out for clues like dark-colored urine, dry mouth, or feelings of lightheadedness.

Understand that activity level and environmental factors play a significant role in influencing your hydration needs. The higher the intensity of your dance routines and warmer the surrounding temperature, the more water loss your body experiences. Adjust your fluid intake accordingly.

8.3. Planning Your Hydration Strategy

To nab the peak-performance trophy, you need to have a detailed strategy for hydration. This should start before you even warm-up for your dance practice.

The American Council on Exercise suggests the following hydration guidelines:

- Pre-exercise: Drink 17 to 20 ounces of water about 2 to 3 hours before your dance workout. Then, consume an additional 8 ounces 20 to 30 minutes before you get moving.

- During exercise: It is recommended to drink 7 to 10 ounces every 10 to 20 minutes throughout your dance session.

- Post-exercise: To replenish any fluid loss during the workout, drink an additional 8 ounces within 30 minutes after dancing, and continue drinking until your urine is light yellow in color.

8.4. Ramp Up with Electrolytes

When you sweat, you're losing more than just water–you're also shedding essential electrolytes like sodium and potassium, key for maintaining your body's balance of fluids. Rehydrate with drinks that contain these electrolytes, especially after intense sessions or performances. Besides sports drinks, natural sources such as coconut water or even a banana can be excellent options.

8.5. Food for Fluids

Your hydrating efforts shouldn't be limited to liquids. Foods can also contribute significantly to maintaining water balance. Fresh fruits and vegetables like watermelon, cucumber, and spinach are excellent choices owing to their high water content.

8.6. Avoid Dance Dehydrators

Certain food and drink, like those high in caffeine and alcohol, can promote dehydration. While a morning cup of coffee or a post-event cocktail isn't entirely prohibited, moderation and ample water compensation is the way to go.

8.7. Unexpected Challenges: Maintaining Hydration in Different Conditions

Whether it is the peak of summertime heat, dry winter months, or simply an air-conditioned studio, various atmospheres affect your hydration needs. Acknowledge this and be proactive in amending your hydration regime to suit these circumstances, ensuring a smooth and effortless dance performance every time.

Hydration is thus not just about drinking water. It is a mindful practice that requires planning, comprehension of body signals, dietary choices, and adaptations to environments. Your dance journey would be incomplete without this vital partner: So, let's put on the music, take a sip, and celebrate hydration's importance on the dance floor. Your pursuit of better fitness and health has found its perfect rhythm.

Chapter 9. Recovery and Restoration: Dance, Nutrition, and the Art of Healing

In the rigorous world of dance and fitness, it's imperative not to underestimate the importance of recovery and restoration. For each rhythmic pump, visceral leap, or gentle sway, your body requires time to heal, digest, and replenish energy. A comprehensive approach to health includes not only diligent attention to movement and nutrition but also devoted care for rejuvenation.

9.1. The Dance of Healing: Understanding the Body's Response to Rhythmic Movement

Dance is more than a delightful form of art and fitness; it's a catalyst for physical healing. Each tap, twirl, and leap pushes your muscles, tendons, and cardiovascular system, leading to micro-tears and energy depletion. While such aftermath may sound worrying, it's nature's brilliant strategy for growth. These micro-tears, when healed, lead to stronger, more resilient muscles – an outcome otherwise known as muscle hypertrophy. Cardiovascular exertion, on the contrary, improves heart and lung function.

The link between dance and progressive healing doesn't end with muscles and heart. Dancing also sparks neuroplasticity – the brain's ability to adapt and rewire itself—reducing cognitive decline and fortifying mental health.

However, these benefits aren't immediate. Dancer's body needs time to repair and adapt. You might experience temporary discomfort, fatigue, or reduced mobility, symptomatic of your body in healing. While discomfort signifies progress, overdoing it can lead to injury or burnout.

9.2. Feeding the Healing: How Nutrition Fuels Restoration

The nutrition-restoration link is as solid as our bones themselves. Literally. The right nutrients can bolster everything from muscle repair to bone density, providing the building blocks your body needs to recover.

Protein, for one, fuels muscle repair. Consuming an ample amount of protein-rich foods such as lean meats, dairy, or plant-based alternatives like lentils and quinoa can do wonders for muscle recovery.

Carbohydrates, too, play a vital role in recovery. Contrary to the vilification they often receive, carbs are crucial energy sources. They restock glycogen stores in muscle cells, the primary source of fuel during intense dance workouts.

Minerals and vitamins are invaluable, performing an array of functions in the body. For instance, Calcium and Vitamin D strengthen bones; Vitamin C supports the immune system and tissue repair, and Omega-3 fats help reduce inflammation post-workouts.

Chapter 10. Hydrate to Regenerate: The Key Role of Water

Water often goes neglected when discussing nutrition, overshadowed by attention-grabbing macro and micronutrients. As the primary component of our bodies, water is critical for every cellular activity, including healing.

Water aids in nutrient transport to the cells, detoxification of metabolic waste produced during workouts and maintenance of body temperature, so crucial for dancers. A hydrated body is an effective body, navigating through the healing process more efficiently.

Chapter 11. Respecting Rest: Sleep as an Ally in Healing

Sleep and rest are fundamental to the body's recovery efforts. They provide your body a cessation from activity, creating an optimal environment for healing and growth.

During deep sleep, the body enters a repair mode. Growth hormone is produced which is instrumental in this process. Moreover, the consolidation of muscle memory, absolutely crucial for dancers, happens during sleep. Prioritizing ample, good-quality sleep alongside nutrition and active healing enhances overall wellness.

Chapter 12. Self-Care Strategies for Dancers

Beyond nutrition and rest, creating a routine of effective self-care will stimulate recovery and protect against wear and tear. This can include foam rolling for tight muscles, yoga for flexibility and relaxation, and mindful meditation to reduce stress and foster mental well-being.

In conclusion, remember that dance, while a powerful tool for physical and mental health, demands respect and care for the body in return. With attention to recovery punctuated with balanced nutrition, hydration, rest, and self-care, you can continue to inch towards better fitness and health, one twirl at a time.

This exhaustive discourse is your map to not just dance your way to health, but thrive in the process. The spotlight's on you; it's time for your dance of healing to begin.

Chapter 13. The Future Dance Floor: Scientific Breakthroughs in Dance and Nutrition

In the kaleidoscopic world of dance, futuristic transformations are brewing. And in the realm of nutrition, new and fascinating discoveries continue to be made, reshaping our understanding of food and health. These two domains—dance and nutrition—are capable of interfacing in exciting new ways, opening up doorways to unexplored dimensions of health and wellness.

13.1. Dance Science: A New Frontier

Advancements in contemporary technology are changing the dance floor landscape. From pedagogic methods to performance analysis, these emerging developments are providing a wealth of insights into the process of dance and our relationship with it. Among these innovations is the world's first 'smart' floor system. The smart floor merges dance and technology, tracking dancers' movements and delivering real-time feedback. This transformative tool presents new opportunities for enhancing dance technique, reducing injury, and augmenting the sensory experience of dance.

Notably, motion capture technology has started playing a crucial role in the scientific study of dance. As the name suggests, this technology captures movement in intricate detail, converting the dancers' dynamism into digital data. The collected data helps dance professionals and researchers evaluate movement patterns, enhance dancers' performance and wellbeing, and develop innovative dance techniques.

On another note, Virtual Reality (VR) is no longer a futuristic concept. A growing number of studios have begun integrating immersive VR environments into their dance routines, opening up exciting possibilities for interaction, learning, and engagement. This includes dancing with virtual partners, experiencing the full immersion of a performing space or challenging oneself by 'dancing' through complex virtual landscapes.

13.2. Evolving Nutritional Paradigms

Parallel to the progress on the dance frontier, nutrition science too has been witnessing breakthroughs that seek to redefine our journey towards an optimally nourished life. The evolving nutritional science focuses on the concept of 'precision nutrition' that strives to provide personalized nutritional advice based on one's genetic makeup, gut microbiome, metabolic responses, and more.

The concept of nutrigenomics explores the relationship between genes, nutrition, and health. It investigates how certain foods might interact with our genes, potentially improving our health and reducing the risk of certain diseases. This opens up new avenues for personalized nutrition plans which can significantly enhance the condition of those who dance regularly, by catering to their unique metabolic needs and recovery plans.

A further impressive breakthrough is the discovery of the gut-brain axis. This axis serves as a communication highway between our gut and our brain, affecting everything from mood to cognitive function. Consuming gut-friendly, easily digestible foods could play a significant role in improving dance performance, from boosting energy levels to enhancing mood and focus.

13.3. Dancing to the Rhythm of Health

Pairing these groundbreaking developments in dance and nutrition science presents a compelling opportunity to promote holistic health. For example, immersing in a VR dance environment after consuming a meal tailored to your genetic profile could maximize your dance efficiency, boost your mood, and aid recovery.

Another interesting aspect is exploring how rhythmic movement impacts digestion and metabolism – a field just beginning to be tapped. Imagine a controlled experiment where participants engage in dance movements choreographed in sync with digestion rates, exploring potential synergies between diet and dance.

13.4. Conclusion

As we stand at the cusp of unprecedented advancements in dance and nutrition, the future dance floor holds immense potential for promoting human health and wellbeing. As increasingly sophisticated technologies and scientific insights permeate both disciplines, the interplay between dance and nutrition is set to become more intricately woven.

These groundbreaking developments herald the dawn of a new era, one that celebrates the confluence of rhythm and nutrition, of movement and health. This fascinating intersection can become the catalyst for a vibrant, synergistic journey towards comprehensive wellness, thereby, remolding our perception of the dance floor – transforming it into a pulsating platform for enhanced health and fitness.

Chapter 14. Your Personalized Dance Nutrition Plan: Choreographing Your Success

Let's cease any further ado and dive right into the process of creating your unique personal dance nutrition plan. By the end of this, you should have a comprehensive understanding and the confidence to choreograph your own dance to success.

14.1. Understanding your Nutritional Needs

The initial yet most important step is to understand your body and its unique needs. Every individual is different, with unique nutritional requirements based on factors such as height, weight, activity levels, and health conditions.

1. **Basal Metabolic Rate (BMR)**: BMR is the amount of energy you burn at rest. That's essentially the number of calories your body needs to perform basic bodily functions like breathing, circulation, and controlling body temperature. You can determine your BMR using various online calculators.

2. **Activity Level**: If you're dancing, your body is in motion and requires more energy than your BMR provides. This additional requirement can be factored in by applying a multiplier to your BMR, known as Physical Activity Level (PAL).

   - Sedentary: If you do little to no exercise, your PAL is 1.2.

   - Lightly active: If you do light exercise 1-3 days per week, your PAL is 1.375.

- Moderately active: If you do moderate exercise 3-5 days per week, your PAL is 1.55.

- Very active: If you do hard exercise 6-7 days per week, your PAL is 1.725.

Your Total Daily Energy Expenditure (TDEE) is then calculated as BMR x PAL. This value gives you a rough estimate of the daily caloric intake required to maintain your current weight.

1. **Nutrient Breakdown**:

   - **Proteins**: They're essential for muscle growth and recovery – both crucial for dancers. The Recommended Dietary Allowance for protein is 46 grams per day for women and 56 grams per day for men.

   - **Fats**: Fats are high-density energy sources. Given the intensity of dance workouts, a healthy amount of fat is necessary. The Dietary Guidelines recommends that 20-35% of your calories come from fat.

   - **Carbohydrates**: Dancers require carbs to maintain energy levels. Aim for complex carbs like whole grains, which release energy slowly and consistently. About 45-65% of your calories should come from carbohydrates.

   - **Vitamins and Minerals**: These are essential for various bodily functions. You can usually achieve the necessary intake through a balanced diet but consult your nutritionist or doctor if you're unsure.

14.2. Designing your Dance Nutrition Plan

With your nutritional requirements in mind, it's time to design your Dance Nutrition Plan. Here are some steps you can follow:

1. **Calculate Daily Calorie Needs**: Using the BMR, PAL, and TDEE knowledge ways we explained earlier, calculate your daily caloric requirements.

2. **Divide Calories Among Meals and Snacks**: Ideally, you should aim for 3 balanced meals and 2-3 healthy snacks per day to keep your energy levels stable.

3. **Balance Macronutrients**: Distribute your daily calorie intake in the ratio of 10-35% proteins, 20-35% fats, and 45-65% carbohydrates.

Example schedule:

|Time|Meal|Protein|Carbohydrates|Fat| |---|---|---|---|---| |8 AM |Breakfast|-|-|-| |11 AM |Snack|-|-|-| |1 PM |Lunch|-|-|-| |4 PM |Snack|-|-|-| |7 PM |Dinner|-|-|-| |Rough Total|-|-|-|-|

Consistently maintaining this schedule ensures that your body gets the required energy and nutrients when it needs them.

14.3. Nutritious Recipes and Snacks

To make your nutrition plan more joyful and less tedious, here are some nutritious recipes and snack ideas that are ideal for dancers:

1. **Protein Pancakes for Breakfast**: These are packed with protein that'll keep your muscles happy and you satiated.

2. **Chicken Salad for Lunch**: This combo offers high-quality protein from the chicken and essential vitamins and minerals from the salad.

3. **Almond and Fruit Snack**: Almonds offer healthy fats and protein, while fruits provide a carb boost and essential micronutrients.

4. **Grilled Fish and Veggies Dinner**: This fulfilling dinner offers a balanced mix of protein from the fish and carbs from the veggies.

14.4. Moving Forward

Remember, consistency is key. Keep dancing, keep eating, and keep enjoying. Track your progress, and don't hesitate to tweak your plan based on your experiences and requirements. Remember that our bodies are unique, and it might take some time to get it all right. Stay patient and stay motivated as you dance your way to better health with Nutritional Harmony.